Feed your Infant for Free and Lose Weight

20 Checklists for New Moms

Bonya Broadnax

authorHOUSE®

AuthorHouse™
1663 Liberty Drive
Bloomington, IN 47403
www.authorhouse.com
Phone: 1 (800) 839-8640

Published by AuthorHouse 12/11/2018

ISBN: 978-1-5462-7025-6 (sc)
ISBN: 978-1-5462-7024-9 (e)

Library of Congress Control Number: 2018914070

Print information available on the last page.

Contents

The goal of this book is to assist you in enjoying your baby. This quick read will be informative, motivate and inspire you as you care for your baby. This book is also formatted for you to return the book and read sections repeatedly as you encounter situations during the first months and years.

Introduction to the Book

Congratulations!! This is a very magical time in your life! Are you pregnant? Thinking about starting a family or adding another baby to your family? Hopefully we can provide you with information to make a smooth transition. Have you just delivered? You have a new baby in your home! Your new bundle of joy is here!! There is so much to discover about your baby! At the same time, allow your body to recover from labor and delivery. Your baby is cuddling, cooing, and gazing up at you. You have some choices to make - Should you breastfeed your baby, how long will you breastfeed, weeks, month, years? Will you supplement your breastfeeding with formula? These are questions new mothers face- it is okay to review these questions weekly or sometimes daily. As you do, refer back to this guide for information and encouragement of the decisions you make. Watch your baby's lips and how the baby holds his mouth and how the baby moves his tongue and sucks his lips. These could be cues for you to take action! Listen to the sounds of the baby- are the sounds wet or are the sounds dry? Can you tell if your baby is hungry or just discovering their lips? Do the sounds get louder and faster? This book is a quick and easy read to guide to encourage healthy bonding between you and your baby from birth to age three!

Being a mother is not about what you gave up to have child, but what you have gained from having one.

---Author Unknown

Chapter 1

Breastmilk is amazing!

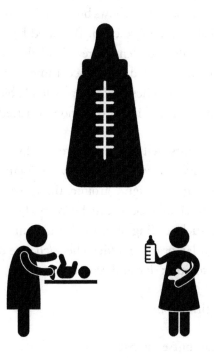

What is exactly in breastmilk?

❖ Lactose

❖ Immunoglobulin(IgA)

❖ Protein

❖ Calories

❖ Fat

❖ Vitamins

❖ Minerals

❖ Digestive Enzymes

❖ Hormones

❖ Antibodies

❖ Lymphocytes

While you care for your baby you may be asked, what are you doing? Why are you nursing your baby? Respond with a few facts! Research shows breastfed babies sleep easier. Breastfed babies are more calm. Breastfed babies have less disease and health problems. Breastfed babies cry less and are less colicly. Breastfed babies according to research, are more smarter than other babies. Breastfed babies show less obesity and less dental issues than non breastfed babies.

How did the nurse tell you to feed your baby?

If you have a newborn, nurse your infant every two hours morning and night, around the clock, 24/7. Your mother, partner or spouse can burp the baby after each feeding. At each feeding offer the breast, nurse baby, burp baby in your lap or on shoulder, check/change diaper, then move baby to other side and repeat.

Positive Affirmations

❑ I can nurse my baby.

❑ I will pace myself with my baby.

- ❑ I can express milk for my baby and give my baby a bottle.
- ❑ I can nurse my baby and/or express milk to prevent engorgement.
- ❑ I can nurse my baby even though my skin is sensitive sometimes.
- ❑ My baby enjoys me holding them.
- ❑ My baby is thriving from my breastmilk
- ❑ I have an adequate milk supply for my baby.
- ❑ I can supplement my breast milk with baby formula.
- ❑ I can call the hospital or doctor's office and make an appointment to see a lactation nurse to assist me.

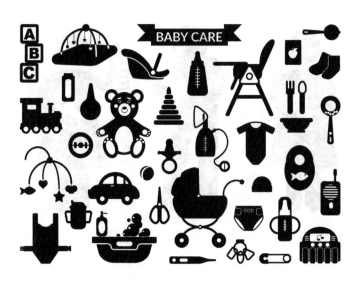

Chapter 2

Breastmilk on Tap 24/7!

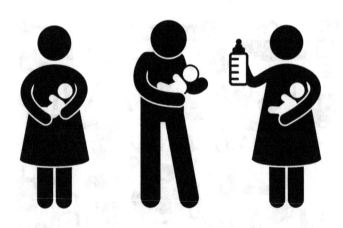

"OMG!, I woke up dripping!" - What to do when your milk comes in!

Let your baby nurse on both sides of your chest to relieve pressure and to satisfy your baby's appetite. Insert absorbent breast pads in your bra for leakage and or express milk with your breast pump. Nurse frequently throughout the day to relieve the fullness felt and to prevent engorgement. Some women express milk with a breast pump after nursing their baby, to develop a milk supply to bottle feed later. You can also nurse your baby on the left side - while you express milk on the right side. Then alternate, nurse on the right side and express on the left breast. Catch the milk when you have a let down! There are nursing pads and soft cups to collect milk under your clothes, in your bra top! Have no fear, your breasts were made to function this way to nourish your newborn! What will you eat while you breastfeed your baby. Let's talk about that later. Breastfeeding uses a lot of resources from the body. During the time you breastfeed, make sure you are feeding YOUR body nutritious meals to restore all the nutrients your body is using to produce milk. During this time you nurse it would be a good time to visit the dentist, the same hormones used and produced in the body for nursing can affect your dental health. Let the dentist monitor any changes in your teeth and gums during this time. Breastfeeding is a commitment. Tell all of your family and friend who surround you that you are planning to nurse and what that means to you and your baby, the private, quiet time and space, it requires and the amount of sleep needed. Your appetite may also change during this time. Frequent thirst and you may need to carry

5

water around throughout the day. What is your weight? Talk to your healthcare provider about what your weight and subsequently what/how much water you need to consume daily while you are nursing.

- ✓ Clothing/fashion
- ✓ Comfort level of spouse/partner/family
- ✓ Ease of handling baby
    - ○ Cradle position
    - ○ Football Hold
    - ○ Laid Back
    - ○ Side Lying
- ✓ Comfort with Body Image
- ✓ Protect, Preserve and Save your Milk Supply

Chapter 3

Around the Clock Feeding, Free No Assembly Required!

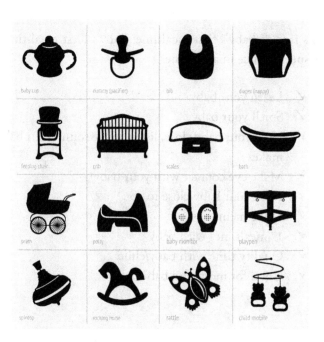

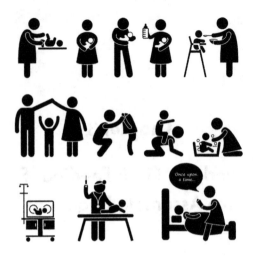

This is your baby's first mealtime! Baby's First meal times are special, once in a lifetime!

- ✓ Learn your baby
- ✓ Smell your baby
- ✓ Hold your baby close, listen to the sound your baby makes
- ✓ Make eye contact with your baby
- ✓ Rock your baby close to you
- ✓ Make memories
- ✓ 1st mealtimes with baby
- ✓ Quality time with baby/child
- ✓ Good for mom and baby

Breastfeeding and Body Image

- ✓ Are you the first to breastfeed in your family?
- ✓ Have you had previous breast surgery or complication?

Whether we like our chest or not - this is why God gave them to us! Value your friends! Value the function of your friends! Get comfortable with your breasts, especially if you want to nurse for a while. Stand in front of the bathroom mirror, look at them, touch them, grab them, pull them, move them to the left or right. No matter if you have small chest or large chest, you do have an adequate milk supply to feed and satisfy your baby. Get use to manipulating your breasts if you will be using a breast pump. The suction from the pump and placing the plastic cups on your chest will give your breasts a workout - like a mammogram - hence nursing and milk production gives you a calorie burn that helps you lose weight. Be hands on!

Breastfeeding is a brief, temporary lifestyle change. Are you high touch, or low touch, when it comes to your breast? Holding, nursing your baby, using a breast pump four to six times a day, then be intimate with your partner at night can be a lot sometimes, but pace yourself and set realistic expectations. Talk to your partner about your physical intimacy needs. Speak to your lactation consultant for more information and support. Don't worry, when your breastfeeding season ends, there are dozens of miracle bras and inserts on the market and you can have plastic surgery to achieve the look you want. What you are giving your baby in your breastmilk is priceless!

The breast is one of the most sexualized part of the body. The breast is a symbol of motherhood. This can be the most time you have ever had an exposed breast. You have to show the nurse in the hospital you can breastfeed. Then you may have nurse in front of your partner, and mother, grandfather, other family, or your older children.

Talk to your family about nursing, nursing overall and talk to your partner/husband about you nursing, their comfort level and nursing in public. For some older children and partners, it may be embarrassing. Talk about the benefits of nursing and your need for privacy and discretion. Practice using a cover or a scarf. If it is your first child, make sure you and your partner are comfortable about nursing in public.

Take it easy at first, nurse at home, and learn how to say something funny to excuse yourself to nurse. Then if your schedule requires you to nurse your baby in public or express milk in public, away from home, create a game plan. You may nurse or express milk in your car or minivan, dressing room in a mall, or family restroom.

- ✓ Try on your nursing bra/top and practice holding the baby or pump with it.
- ✓ Walk through packing, unpacking your pump on the go & storing your milk in a cold pack tote on the go!
- ✓ Practice using your diaper bag, tucking away your nursing cover, & changing diapers on the go.
- ✓ What items can you keep in the car to help care for your baby?
- ✓ Practice speaking up and saying "I'll be back in a minute" - diaper changing time, or I have to go pump".

Chapter 4

Breastmilk, Not much needed!

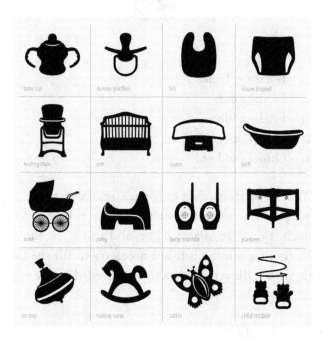

baby cup | dummy (pacifier) | bib | diaper (nappy)
feeding chair | crib | scales | bath
pram | potty | baby monitor | playpen
spintop | rocking horse | rattle | child mobile

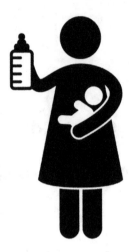

- ☐ Relax
- ☐ Bonding Time
- ☐ Feeding cues
- ☐ Feeding Blitz
- ☐ Size of baby stomach
- ☐ Ounces add up!

Your baby stomach is only the size of cherry the day she was born, the size of a walnut by day 3, by day 5 the stomach is the size of an apricot, and an egg by the end of the first month. So it is not necessary to fill the large bottle with milk yet!! Only a little is needed? How much exactly?

Expressed Milk Required:

Newborn	1-3oz	8-12oz a day
3w-3ms	3-4oz	32oz a day

3m-6m	4-8oz	24-32oz a day
6-9m	6-8oz	32oz a day
9-12m	7-8oz	24-32oz a day

To Thaw Frozen Milk

❖ Sit in fridge
❖ Sit in warm water
❖ Swirl, don't shake
❖ Do not microwave
❖ Do not heat up or add to storage bag!

This is your baby - your blood extension of you. Your genetic match that you created!

By nursing your baby, you continue the physical connection from the womb.

✓ Spending time together
✓ Skin to skin contact
✓ Comfort by natural mom

This baby is your 24/7 love! The baby likes you, likes how you smell, laugh! Your baby wants to be around you morning, noon, and night. The baby likes your hair, clothes, how you dress and walk!! There goes my mommy!

You are your baby mama! Your Baby wants you!

Why am I doing this? Because it is good for me and the baby!

✓ Emotionally and physically
✓ Strengthen the bond between you and your child

13

- ✓ Nursing benefits you and your baby!
- ✓ Post partum healing of mom
- ✓ Continue baby growth
- ✓ Calorie burn,
- ✓ Uterus cramp to decrease flattening your stomach
- ✓ Sleep ease
- ✓ Less crying
- ✓ Obesity prevention
- ✓ Dental benefits

You are #1 to your Baby!

The Baby likes you just the way you are! You have the perfect hair, skin, body type, you smell good to them. Your children like your voice, want to hear you talk, laugh, sing. Your baby looks for you— wants you when you leave the room. You baby misses you when you leave them! These are some of the things you think about when you date someone and when you are out with your adult friends, but it is different with your children. Babies crave their mother, sometimes more than anyone else. You are A, number #1 to your baby. Your baby wants you to stay well and be healthy! Your baby wants to look, gaze into your eyes everyday!

You can do it! Read and reread the affirmations!

- ♥ My baby loves and accepts me for me!
- ♥ My body is a temple, I will love and care for my body.
- ♥ Now that I am a mother, I will be careful of what I eat and drink.

♥ I can lose weight and maintain a healthy weight so I can lead an active lifestyle!

♥ I choose long life for myself and my family so I choose to lead a healthy lifestyle.

♥ I care for myself so I can care for my baby!

For this child I have prayed and the Lord has granted the desires of my heart!
-Sammuel 1:27

Chapter 5

Create a Lunch Milk Station!

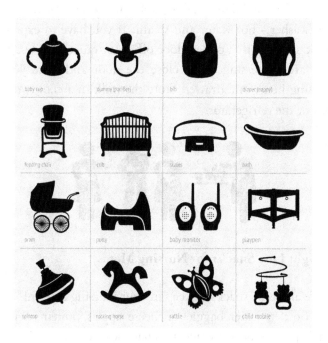

baby cup	dummy (pacifier)	bib	diaper (nappy)
feeding chair	crib	scales	bath
pram	potty	baby monitor	playpen
spintop	rocking horse	rattle	child mobile

Organize your Baby Nursing Area

Keep all nursing items/ things (pump, plastics, shield, milk storage bags) clean and sanitized. Be careful with storage of your baby/nursing items in your gym bag. Store them in a separate clean Ziploc bag. Wash your hands thoroughly before you open the bag and handle the items.

Keep the kitchen countertops clean. Leave cleaning supplies, wipes, solutions in spray bottle on high shelves out of the way of children. Use wipes to swipe across surfaces in kitchen - the kitchen table, high chair, toddler seat. This is also the time to use the top rack, sanitizing cycle of your dishwasher - hot water and steam. If you have to express milk at work, in a closed door office, or quiet cubicle and you are expressing milk, close the door and store your nursing items in a drawer. Store the milk in a cooler, tote bag or the refrigerator.

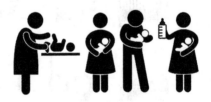

Weight Loss Snacks for Nursing Moms

Here are some snacks to keep in your Nursing Station:

Bottled Water, baggies of cheese, apples, protein energy bars, peanut butter crackers, chapstick, and hand lotion Stash goodie bags in car/office/home. Refill bags after trip to grocery store.

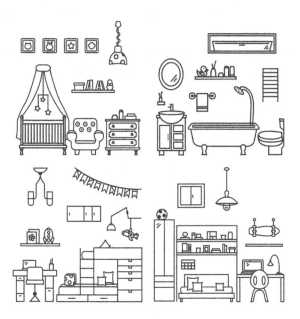

How do you create a space for you and your baby? Visit kids stores, catalogs and magazines. Identify the space or room that will be the baby's area. Measure the walls, doorways, and windows and carry the measurements with you when you go shopping to look for items. Look at fabric, and paint chips, notice the sunlight in the room and decide on a shade of color for the bedroom and bathroom. Check out the many different kits available in the fabric, arts and crafts store to make window treatments!

✓ *I can nourish myself and my baby by creating, using and going to the nursery area/corner to rest and connect with my baby.*
✓ *I can create a caring and safe space for me and my baby.*

- ✓ *I can create an environment safe for me and my family to grow.*
- ✓ *I can nourish myself by practicing being 100% present and attentive while nursing the baby.*

God Bless this Home with Great Love
Bless the Walls and Corners Above
Bless the Doors that Open Wide
Welcoming Happiness to All
Who Enter Inside

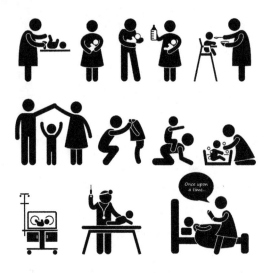

Create Functional Baby Area

Decorate, make the room corner functional - place nursing/gliding chair close to window for sunlight. Chair is excellent for rocking, reading nursing, and napping. Decided to have bookcase in room to share children's book and baskets of photos and albums and music, so the toddler and young child can access the basket and shelves as a "self serve, music, books, and games".

If you are introducing a baby into a family that already has children, plan activity areas for every room of the house. Keep toys and books accessible wherever they are - puzzles for entertainment while I prepared the food/meals. Small table and chairs, kids sized table and chairs so the kids could enjoy sliding the chair out from under the table. Even the refrigerator I cleaned the bottom shelf so when standing in front of the opened door, the toddler would/could just reach for snacks or water on the bottom shelf.

★ Sunlight
★ Bookshelf
★ Toy chest
★ Comfortable seating
★ Childproof
★ Kids sized table/chairs

Babies and Toddlers make noise, cry a lot and are sometimes messy! Remember they are just growing and expressing their needs and feelings! Love them anyway!!

Make a joyful noise unto the Lord, all the earth: make a loud noise, and rejoice, and sing praise. Psalm 98:4

Create an Area for Yourself, Mom and Baby

Some people choose to work with an Interior Designer, what is the advantage?

Sometimes all you need is two consultation visits with the designer, especially if you are a "hands on" crafty type person. If you already have an idea of what the space should look like, put it on paper. Create a nursery plan with hand drawings and color chips/scheme to share with the designer. You can create the nursery you see in the magazines, it starts with you!! Have the interior designer come to your home, share your plans with him or her. He like my plans and he shared with me information on issues to think about in planning, using certain type of materials in the room, and how the room will fit into the overall decor and flow of the house.

Interior Designers can offer you exclusive access, better sourcing, information on products, care of fabric and surface areas, and of course new ideas, and referrals to other experts/contractors to fit your needs and budget.

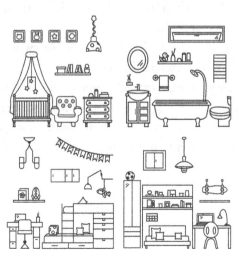

A Few Childproofing Home Tips from NAEYC Safety Checklist - National Association for the Education of Young Children

- ✓ Place covers over the electrical outlets, especially in open areas where baby/kids crawl and play
- ✓ Clear items off coffee table/console table, when baby starts pulling up on table, we don't want anything to fall on them
- ✓ Cover sharp edges of coffee tables, or countertops
- ✓ Lock away cleaning supplies, clean when they are asleep and place back behind lock at night

Where will you exercise?

- ✓ TV Monitor
- ✓ Mat and space to stretch
- ✓ Safe storage space to keep dumb bells and exercise equipment
- ✓ Exercise when baby is sleep, early morning or light stretch at night
- ✓ If baby wakes, identify bassinet or swing to place them into exercise for ten minutes
- ✓ Keep gym bag in car with running shoes or walking shoes
- ✓ Identify an area to walk/run with a stroller in your community near your home, work, or school.
- ✓ Read, listen to music, mediate in your space

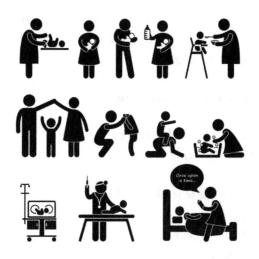

Creating a Baby Cozy Corner

While you nurse, it is imperative to position yourself and baby at the most ergonomic position possible. Use pillows and sit in comfortable yet firm chair. Gather everything you need before you start nursing. Create a "nursing station" for yourself and your baby. Create one for work and at home and in the car. Your nursing station could include a chair, glider, end table, lamp, water, a snack "fruit" snack, towel napkin. Keep a soft robe with pocket where you keep a tube of lotion or chapstick. You could include music- a special playlist, or one of the baby's tops or blanket to promote let down. Consistency is key. Once you identify the best time and place to nurse, Gather all of your materials - your robe, breast pump, water, quiet music, baby lovey toy. Milk let down should come easily and naturally - almost systematic. If you baby has a sibling have book game, puzzle or toy to share with the sibling to sit, talk, sing and bond together as a family or let them. This is very important family bonding time. What you read, the activities you play are things they can do later as they grow.

Items for your Baby Cozy Corner

- ✓ Soft Fuzzy Robe with deep pockets
- ✓ Chair/glider
- ✓ Sofa
- ✓ Table -close to electrical outlet
- ✓ Lamp
- ✓ Playlist/Speaker
- ✓ Bassinet/Cot

Table

- ✓ Pump
- ✓ Water Bottle
- ✓ Speaker
- ✓ Book/Toy
- ✓ Fruit/Protein Snack for Mom
- ✓ Diaper/Onesie
- ✓ Smartphone for Timer & Journal/Pic Apps

Sofa/Chair

- ✓ Extra pillow for support
- ✓ Book/Magazine
- ✓ Soft Towel/Blanket
- ✓ Diaper/Onesie

Fuzzy Robe Deep Pocket
   Chapstick
   Cream/Lotion
   Pads

"Kick off your shoes, put on your fuzzy robe, socks and relax!"

Relax so baby can relax and open wide for a painless latch on. You may want to stretch before you sit down to nurse and /or after you nurse. Beware of your posture after you nurse. Position the baby to move and be close to you - bring the baby close to you. Do not slouch down to the baby - Roll your shoulders back and strengthen your arms, shoulder and upper back with light weights. Some women want to multi-task when nursing. Remember nursing is a special bonding time with you and your baby. But when you have to entertain a toddler while you nurse be ready to have baby in one arm and a pillow and have the other arm free to play a game, read books, give hugs. feed children, work your iPad, sent a text. But don't forget about the baby. If you must work/entertain for a minute then gaze back down at your baby. Once you have gotten into the routine of nursing relax while you nurse. Get to know yourself and your energy level. If you have had a long day, when it is time to nurse, nurse with your "feet up", stretch your legs out, snuggle with the baby. If you are sleepy - be careful to position the baby so it can nurse but anchor a pillow underneath your arm and the baby so if you dose off to sleep and your arm relaxes the baby is still safe in your arms.

Take off your work uniform, suit, and slide on your favorite robe to snuggle with your baby. A thick, soft robe with pockets are the best for nursing moms. Add a hook to the back of the bathroom door and keep it there! Enjoy your nursing experience. Make nursing hip and trendy!! If you decide to nurse in public be prepared for praise and criticism. When you hear criticism, smile and educate. Many people do not know the benefits of breastfeeding for the mother, great nutrition for the baby and bonding experience for the whole family. Also, if you are sensitive to the comments become a "researcher", pretend you are surveying people, and notice who the negative comments come from. Let the criticism slide off your back. Visit a La Leche League meeting and surround yourself around other nursing moms or moms who did nurse their children.

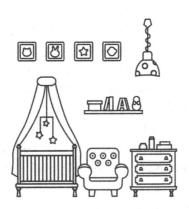

Chapter 6

Breastfeed Longer!

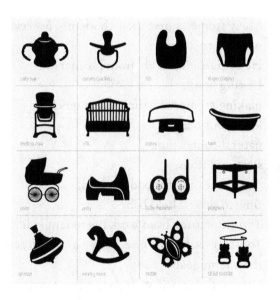

When are you going back to work?

- ✓ Keep a calendar
- ✓ Reward yourself for milestones
- ✓ Check your relationship with your partner
- ✓ Check your lifestyle
- ✓ Exclusively pump?
- ✓ Extended breastfeeding?
- ✓ Do you have milk stored in freezer?

Why breastfeed longer?

- ❑ Many women nurse their children ~ 6 weeks to ~3 months, to 2 years
- ❑ Helps transition body from pregnancy
- ❑ Lasting bond,
- ❑ making memories - time passes quickly,
- ❑ learn your baby,
- ❑ natural connection,
- ❑ start traditions,
- ❑ natural healing for body to heal,
- ❑ time to sit and hold baby
- ❑ Transition time from work life to family life
- ❑ You may want to nurse longer as you reach your short term goals.
- ❑ Surround yourself with supportive nursing moms and a plan to pump at your workplace
- ❑ motherhood rite of passage
- ❑ good for mother

Nighttime Nursing Lullaby for you and Your Baby

This is a traditional lullaby, you can substitute mama for pappa!

> Hush, little baby, don't say a word
> Papa's going to buy you a mockingbird.
>
> If that mockingbird won't sing.
> Papa's going to buy you a diamond ring.
>
> If that diamond ring turns brass,
> Papa's going to buy you a looking glass.
>
> If that looking glass gets broke.
> Papa's going to buy you a billy goat.

When you go back to work, reconnect with your baby at night.

- ✓ Co sleep with Baby
- ✓ Beside the bed co-sleeper or bassinet
- ✓ Convertible Crib
- ✓ Twin beds in room
- ✓ Queen bed with side rails
- ✓ Keep room dark
- ✓ Soft music

Chapter 7

Latch Love -There is a Pump for you!

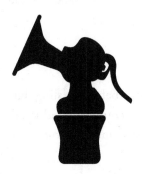

The breast pump market is exploding with new gadget? Which one is best for you? Which one is covered by insurance?

- ❑ Read reviews and watch Facebook/YouTube videos
- ❑ Attend support group for recommendations from other moms
- ❑ Get references from doctor/nurse/lactation nurses
- ❑ Battery Operated?
- ❑ Double Electric?

❑ Manual Hand Pump?
❑ Where will you use the Pump (home, car, office)?
❑ How often will you use the pump?

What to Wear When Expressing Milk

★ Invest in a full length mirror so you can see your full outfit!
★ Cami Top, Elastic Waist Bands, Separates Top and Skirt, Top and Pants
★ Layered sweaters, ponchos,
★ Comfortable shoes, ballerina flats, wedge heels, low heels

Baby Wearing

By wearing your baby in a sling, hands free, improves, preserves posture, encourages bonding, free movement walk with baby, with baby in sling you can hold toddlers hand or push stroller

❑ Baby sling
❑ Baby Wrap
❑ Nursing Cover and Sling
❑ Padding baby wrap
❑ Check your posture

The Absolute Necessities

- Breast Pump/Storage bags
- Pillow
- Cold pack tote for milk
- Sippy cup
- Nursing pads
- Baby Sling
- Nursing Bra top/camisole
- Baby onesie or toy
- Diapers

Stages of Milk

- ✓ Colostrum day 3 to 4
- ✓ High fat concentration -6weeks
- ✓ High in calories & brain development-3mos
- ✓ Protein -6mos
- ✓ Calories -12mos

Prevent Engorgement

- ❖ Manual Hand Pump (MPH)
- ❖ Hand express milk
- ❖ Warm water bath

Infant Baby Feeding Cues

- ✓ Rooting
- ✓ Hand to mouth movement
- ✓ Turning head

Exclusive Pumpers and Schedule

- Every 2 to 3 hours
- 20 minutes sessions
- 6 to 8 times a day from baby age 3 months to 6 months

Pump Schedule

6 am

9 am

12 noon

3 pm

6 pm

9 pm

12 midnight

3 am

Avoid Foods

✓ Caffeine (soda, coffee, chocolate)
✓ Alcohol
✓ Cabbage, Cauliflower
✓ Spicy Foods

Breastmilk Boosters

✓ Mothers Milk Tea
✓ Fenugreek
✓ Lactation Cookies
✓ Lactation Smoothies

Chapter 8

Hydrate & Moisturize!

Body Care

It takes at least 18 months to return to normal following the birth of a child. Remember to moisturize from the inside out. Drink plenty of water because the body is made up of 70% water and your body is producing milk. Carry your water bottle, buy water in bulk or subscribe to a home water service. Choose an all natural moisturizer to slather on your body daily. Pay attention to your feet, knees, elbows- you know the rough spots. Do not use lotion on your chest, if you do, wipe off two hours before you express milk or nurse. No soap is required, nor lotion. Be careful, some products could dry the sensitive area/skin on your chest. While the baby sleeps is a good time to turn your bathroom into a spa, take a quick bath, shampoo your hair, groom yourself, remove stray hair. See how much you can do. Uplift your mood by caring for your hair and skin. Choose to wear a light scent or perfume on your ankles away from the baby. Choose to wear a light natural deodorant. Pat your deodorant product under your arm, that way you do not use too much but you are covered. Your baby may place their hand under your arm while you nurse. You want to protect your baby from any and all chemicals.

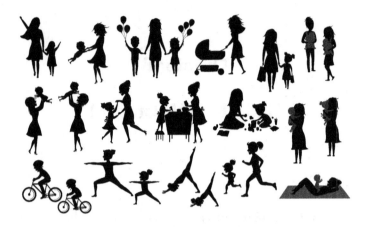

Your body produces breastmilk and it drains from other areas of your body, leaving the skin dry! Eat up and drink up!

- ★ Drink water
- ★ Use lotion or oils
- ★ Follow daily/weekly routine
- ★ Avoid oil, cream or lotion on chest area
- ★ Treat yourself to a Mani/Pedi
- ★ Keep lotion in car, bag, work space
- ★ Keep water bottle on hand

Hydrate and Cleanse

- ✓ Water, Green Tea, Hot Tea, with Citrus Fruit Slices
- ✓ Lactation Tea, Calming Tea but

Chapter 9

Calling All Family and Friends!

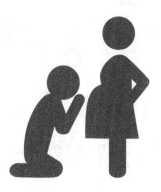

Your family is growing! The pregnancy could have been planned or a surprise! Planning a baby shower, moving closer to loved ones, having a baby around the holiday can bring the family together.

- ✓ What is your parenting philosophy?
- ✓ Do you have a birth plan?
- ✓ Who will be on the babysitting list?
- ✓ What do you want to do different with this baby?

✓ Starting new family traditions
✓ Who is on the babysitting list?

Have some OMG Moments - share medical history and child rearing wisdom at family dinner, baby shower!

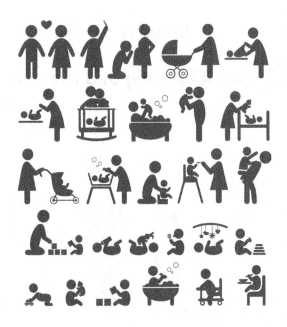

Playing Babydoll - Being a Mommy Role Model

Nursing is a memorable experience that you and your child will have and enjoy the rest of their lives. Five year olds who have nursed until the age of two sometimes remember snuggling with their mothers in the glider, sitting in bed, and riding in the baby sling. They also want to nurse their babydoll. For some, storytime started while nursing and when it is continued it can be a family tradition and wonderful memory that continues. Some mothers find later they are being a role model to their older children, cousins, and neighbors by showing them how to mother or care for an infant.

Did you play with Barbie Dolls? Did you play with Baby Alive? Did you name your real child after the name of your favorite baby doll? Some women do! Well, when you have your own infant, it is time to play classic babydoll - you get to bathe her, change her clothes, change her diaper, wrap her in a blanket, and hold her to your chest, feed her and burp her. This play time with your baby is what some women dream of!! Be aware other women are watching you. Unknowingly, you could become a role model for a little girl, or teenager, or college student, or babysitter who has not seen another woman care for an infant. Some women have never seen another woman breastfeed a baby. You are role modeling, showing others how to care for a baby.

Are you the first mommy in your group? Are you the first mommy parenting your baby differently? Are you the only mommy in your group nursing your baby, don't be discouraged! Find a mother's support group in your community or online!

Be strong and courageous! Do not be afraid of them! The Lord your God will go ahead of you. He will neither fail nor nor forsake you! Deuteronomy 31:6

When it's time to go back to work...

Don't be afraid of criticism. Find your level of mothering and attachment. Be honest with yourself and your partner. Your mental health is paramount during this time of transitioning, adding a new baby in your life.

- ☐ Girls Night Out
- ☐ Take a part time job
- ☐ Work from Home Job
- ☐ Hire a trustworthy Babysitter/Nanny
- ☐ Drop In Daycare
- ☐ Weekend Trip without Kids
- ☐ Wean gently while you are away
- ☐ Barter babysitting with mommy friends, neighbors
- ☐ Schedule a routine weekly spa trip
- ☐ Schedule a half day or full day at the Spa or salon

Chapter 10

Making Liquid Gold Last!

Why should you store your mother's milk? So other family and friends can feed and bond with the baby, and it gives you free time.

The use of your stored Mother's Milk yields more time with grandma or vacation/date night with your partner, family, friend bonding time; they can offer the baby a bottle, or you can donate your milk. Even when you stop nursing your baby, you can continue to store your milk until you stop producing milk or wean. Talk to your doctor about how to properly freeze and thaw breastmilk. Also, speak to your nurse or lactation consultant about donating unused frozen milk. Wash your hand thoroughly before handling "thawed" breastmilk or "defrosted" breastmilk. Make sure the baby bottle is clean and sanitized before filling it with milk. It is worth the investment of purchasing the microwave baby bottle sanitizer to sanitize all plastic nursing and feeding equipment. Save the milk you express. Store the milk-freeze it for use later. This milk, mother's milk can be used with the father and/or babysitter so you can have a few hours to yourself shopping or at the relaxing at the salon. More on milk storage below.

Here are the FDA and Centers for Disease Control and Prevention guidelines for Milk Storage:

Deep Freeze BM	12 months
Fridge Freezer	4 months
Fridge	4 days
Kitchen Counter	4 hours
Used bottle	2 hours

NEVER refreeze breastmilk after its been thawed. Once it's thawed, use that day!

To thaw frozen Breastmilk

- Sit in fridge!
- Sit in Warm water!
- Swirl, don't shake!
- Do not add anything to it!
- Do not microwave!
- Do not warm-up nor heat up breastmilk!

Chapter 11

Supplement your feedings!

♦ Start solids when child is 6 to 8 months
♦ Identify which formula to use
♦ Watch for allergies
♦ Save formula for babysitter, daycare
♦ Watch for change in bowel movements

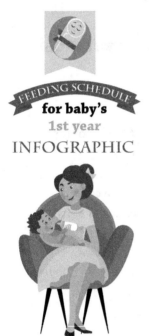

FEEDING SCHEDULE
for baby's
1st year
INFOGRAPHIC

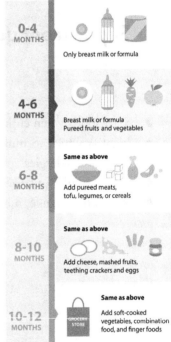

0-4 MONTHS

Only breast milk or formula

4-6 MONTHS

Breast milk or formula
Pureed fruits and vegetables

6-8 MONTHS

Same as above

Add pureed meats,
tofu, legumes, or cereals

8-10 MONTHS

Same as above

Add cheese, mashed fruits,
teething crackers and eggs

10-12 MONTHS

Same as above

Add soft-cooked
vegetables, combination
food, and finger foods

Chapter 12

Clean everything!

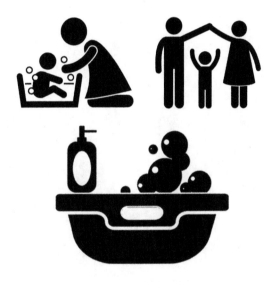

More CDC and FDA guidelines on how to clean Breast Pump parts:

- Clean hands and pump bottles
- Check pump instruction manual
- Top rack of dishwasher

- Wash all breast pump parts that come in contact with the breastmilk, bottles, valves, and breast shields
- Wash with warm water and liquid dishwashing soap
- Let tubing air dry
- Wipe down breast pump motor with soft towel or cloth
- Let pump parts air dry-assemble and store

Chapter 13

Superfoods for Mom and Baby!

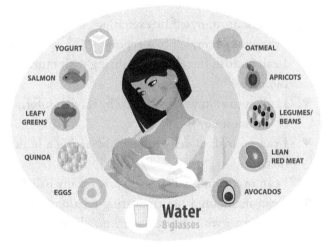

SUPERFOODS
FOR BREASTFEEDING

YOGURT

SALMON

LEAFY GREENS

QUINOA

EGGS

OATMEAL

APRICOTS

LEGUMES/ BEANS

LEAN RED MEAT

AVOCADOS

Water
8 glasses

How can you nourish yourself? I can nourish myself by eating a healthy diet staying physically active, and getting adequate sleep! We all know input influences output - what you digest can influence your energy and mood! Fill your diet with fruit and veggies and hydrate! Drink your eight glasses of water. Eat fresh and whole fruit and veggies whenever possible. Talk to your doctor about taking a multivitamin and consuming other nutritional supplements, juices, meal replacements shakes, and smoothies. Commit to eating high energy nutritious foods, while you nurse. What is your experience with diets? Do you have experience completing a weight loss program, or experience changing your diet due to digestive issues. Draw on your past diet experiences to prepare more meals and snacks at home, in your kitchen, to maintain your appropriate weight and sustain your energy and good mood!

Add your own Positive Affirmations! You can do it!

- ♥ I can nourish myself by exercising
- ♥ I can nourish myself by sleeping
- ♥ I can nourish myself by socializing with other new moms!
- ♥ I can nourish myself and baby by staying informed of the latest news!
- ♥ I can nourish myself and baby by eating a healthy diet!
- ♥ I can overcome challenges to care for my baby!
- ♥ I can maintain a healthy caring relationship with my partner while I care for my new baby!

Get it new mom! Be encouraged!

Eat Superfoods - Gives you Energy - and Lose Weight!

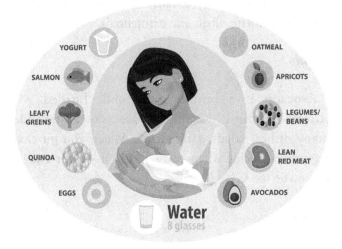

SUPERFOODS
FOR BREASTFEEDING

YOGURT

SALMON

LEAFY
GREENS

QUINOA

EGGS

OATMEAL

APRICOTS

LEGUMES/
BEANS

LEAN
RED MEAT

AVOCADOS

Water
8 glasses

Superfoods

What is a superfood? A superfood is a category of food that is high in nutrients. By eating superfoods, make every bite count, don't waste your time with processed food that doesn't have much nutrients. Whenever possible, eat foods as close to its raw, whole state. I prefer raw fruits and veggies in a salad, smoothies, or steamed, preserving the essence of the food. Below are five popular superfoods. Each meal contains one or more superfoods. Review the suggestions, choose your favorite to add to your meal repertoire!

Greens

Leafy green vegetables are key to a healthy diet. Leafy greens are filled with vitamins C, K, iron and calcium. Of the varieties of leafy greens, the top five filled with antioxidants, folate, fiber, and carotenoids.

Avocado

Avocado is a buttery superfood. Loaded with nutrients vitamin B, K. Slices of avocado can be added t many dishes, salads, sandwiches. When you purchase an avocado, decide when you will use it—right away or later in the week.

Salmon

Salmon is one of the more nutrient dense fish. Because of it popularity, the price of salmon has been reduced and it can be found in more easy to use forms—such as salmon burgers and mal portion salmon filets. Omega-fatty acids, protein, and vitamin D are found in salmon. The dishes listed below in the meal plan capitalize on how convenient salmon s to prepare. Another nutrient dense fish is sardines. Sardines are high in vitamin B, phosphorus, and calcium, and low in mercury.

Berries

Some of the popular superfoods berries are acai berries, blueberries, and Goji. Including blueberries in salads and oatmeal for breakfast is a popular practice. Smoothies are another good place to drop berries.

Nuts

Which nut is your favorite? Almonds, walnuts, or pecans? The almond is a versatile nut. It can be consumed in many forms - raw or via liquid as in almond milk. Almond milk contains Vitamin E and C and many people use it in their morning cereal instead of cow's milk. Be careful, some people gain weight with almond milk. Walnuts are a popular choice of nut and is thought to be an excellent brain food. Walnuts are filled with Vitamin E, and omega-3 fatty acids. I also include sunflower seeds in this category. Add just a handful to your salad, for a crunch!! Nuts can be in different forms - sliced, crumbled, whole, and roasted.

Below are some meal suggestions. These foods and meals are full of antioxidants, omega-3s, and probiotics. Food is cooked with olive oil, seasoned with onion and garlic.

Breakfast Ideas

- ✓ Breakfast Burrito with Egg and Avocado
- ✓ Oatmeal (Chia, Flaxseeds) with berries, walnuts, and cinnamon, with green tea
- ✓ Spinach, egg, cheese omelet with with fresh squeezed citrus juice
- ✓ Whole grain cereal with rice/almond milk
- ✓ Veggie Frittata
- ✓ Bowl of cantaloupe chunks and blueberries

Lunch

- ✓ California Club Sandwich
- ✓ Turkey Avocado
- ✓ Vegetable and Cheese Quiche and Salad
- ✓ Green Salad with Sunflower Seeds
- ✓ Chinese Chicken Salad
- ✓ Beans and Rice with Steamed Vegetable
- ✓ Nut Butter Toast on Whole Grain Bread and Fruit
- ✓ Southwest Taco Salad
- ✓ Veggie Burger/Sandwich (add Tofu or Sprouts) and Salad

Dinner

- ✓ Cheese Quesadillas
- ✓ Fish or Seafood Tacos
- ✓ Grilled Salmon with Green Vegetable/Salad
- ✓ Bok Choy Stir Fry Seafood and Vegetables over Brown Rice or Noodles
- ✓ Steamed Kale with Brown Rice or Quinoa
- ✓ Soup and Salad with Vegetable and Whole Grain
- ✓ Masaman Curry Chicken
- ✓ Skinless, Boneless, BBQ Chicken Breast

Packasnack for the Morning or evening

- ★ Yogurt with Fruit and Nuts
- ★ Guacamole or Hummus and Whole Grain Crackers and Carrots
- ★ Fruit, Cheese and Whole Grain Crackers

★ Half a grapefruit
★ Pomegranate

What are you favorite nutritious foods? What are your favorite fruits and vegetables? Introduce these first to your baby!! Introduce these foods to your baby through your breastmilk.

Notice how baby reacts to the milk following nursing session - which food they may like or dislike. Notice what foods you eat and how your baby responds to them. The foods you eat flavor your milk for the baby. Within minutes after eating certain foods you may tell if and how your baby will respond. As you know, during the time of nursing and breastfeeding, obtain from using drugs and alcohol. If you decide t have a sip of wine, choose the amount and time when you will drink. Wait 2 hours before expressing or pumping milk.

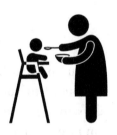

Introducing Solid Foods

What foods should I introduce first?
Speak to your pediatrician. Dilute some fruit and vegetables with water or breastmilk.
Introduce the Colors of the Rainbow

- ❖ Yellow/Orange - Sweet Potatoes, Carrots. Squash, spotted Bananas
- ❖ Red- Baked Apple
- ❖ Blue - Blueberry
- ❖ Green -peas, kale, swiss chard

Setting the Table for Meal Time

- ★ Tabletop decorating
- ★ High Chair
- ★ Daylight/Dim Light

Food Allergies

What allergies do you and dad have? Keep a food diary of what you introduced to your baby. Introduce one food for a few days to make sure there is not an allergy. Notice any skin rashes, vomiting, and change in bowel movements. Call your doctor if there is an allergic reaction. Was your baby allergic to any infant formulas? What food allergies run in the family? Speak to your doctor about what first foods are best for your baby and the best timing and age to introduce them. Many suggest offering banana first.

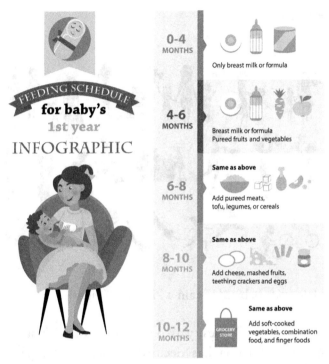

FEEDING SCHEDULE for baby's 1st year INFOGRAPHIC

0-4 MONTHS
Only breast milk or formula

4-6 MONTHS
Breast milk or formula
Pureed fruits and vegetables

Same as above
6-8 MONTHS
Add pureed meats,
tofu, legumes, or cereals

Same as above
8-10 MONTHS
Add cheese, mashed fruits,
teething crackers and eggs

Same as above
10-12 MONTHS
Add soft-cooked
vegetables, combination
food, and finger foods

Positive Affirmations (You can do it! Be Encouraged!!)

✓ I can gently transition my baby from breastfeeding to solid foods.

✓ I can buy and/or prepare nutritious health food for my baby.

✓ Meal time with my baby is a calm, comfortable, pleasant time to share, connect, laugh, and eat nutritious foods!

Exercise

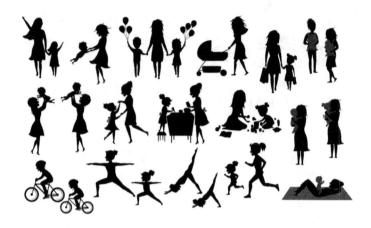

Help your Baby Maintain a Healthy Weight!

Childhood obesity is one of the issues First Lady Michelle Obama has decided to target as a part of her First Lady's initiative. Let's Move is her program to promote and motivate children, parents, childcare workers, and health care providers to encourage children and families to be more physically active at home and school. Let's Move also provides direction on nutrition. Let's Move promotes more healthy eating. Eating more veggies and low fat, low sugar foods. The ChooseMyPlate icon continues in the tradition of the old food pyramid on giving direction what food groups should be used, setting at the table-sharing meals and now portion size. Portion size has been shown to contribute to overeating, increase calories which leads to obesity.

Lose Weight Naturally after the Baby

- ✓ Drink Water
- ✓ Eat Clean Superfoods
- ✓ Jumpstart your Weight Loss with Breastfeeding!
- ✓ Stay Positive
- ✓ Carry nutritious snacks with you!
- ✓ Stroller Walks

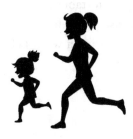

- ❖ How many calories you burn from breastfeeding
- ❖ Talk to your doctor about taking a multivitamin supplement
- ❖ Eat fortified foods - vitamins D, C, Iron, Folic Acid and Iodine

Did you exercise while you were pregnant? Took a prenatal exercise class? It is important to stay active during this time. Exercising and increasing your heart rate will promote a better blood flow through the body and assist you with let down during nursing. However, vigorous exercising may not fit your style or activity during this time. Tai Chi or Yoga may be just what you need to practice while the baby sleeps. There are a number of Yoga, Tai Chi, and Pilates videos on the market that would allow you to exercise, stretch, and tone your body during the first couple of weeks following birth. It is important to follow your body - be gentle with your body - do not force your body into certain moves if it is not ready yet. Listen to your body.

Many women wear belts around their waist while they exercise or while they run their errands around town, throughout the day. The belt gently places and pulls the stomach in place, training the tummy to be flat!! It is important to be as comfortable as possible while you nurse. But one way to assist yourself in keeping good posture during this time is wearing a waist belt a few hours a day for extra support.

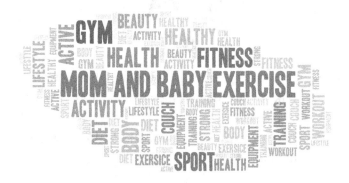

Chapter 14

Saving the Family Dollar!

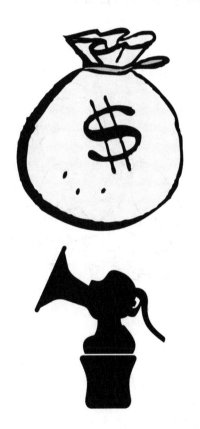

Feed your Infant for Free and Lose Weight

Breastfeeding is free compared to formula feeding! The cost is time!

→ Invest in a pump
→ Nursing bra/tops
→ Use your pump, hands, save a dollar
→ Online Shopping
→ Coupon Apps
→ Shop on schedule
→ Visit Health Department
→ Moms pump & Hand express to save a dollar (MPH)

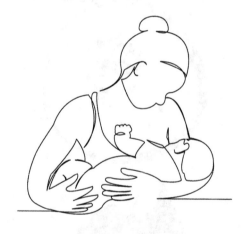

Chapter 15

Mama Bear –Snuggling with the Baby!

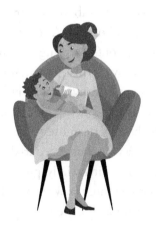

- ❖ Special bonding time with your baby
- ❖ Take pictures
- ❖ Sing songs
- ❖ Play music
- ❖ Read stories
- ❖ Have a conversation with your Baby

Bond with your Baby! Show Your Love! Latch Love!

Have you heard of the Five Love Languages? How do you express your love to your partner, other family members and friends? The Five Love Languages was written by Gary Chapman. They are Words of Affirmation, Acts of Service, Affection, Quality Time, Gifts. You may want to share the book Five Love Languages with your partner. Let's add a sixth love language, Latch Love.

Your baby is a new person, how are you going to love this child? How were you loved? The new baby is a chance to do things differently. It can be a do over if this is your second or third child. Because this is a new beginning, you may want to talk to a counselor about any unresolved issues you may have from your childhood. Also join a parenting group or read a few books about parenting, discipline, and how to better communicate with this new person - a new bundle of joy. Seek out other healthy, supportive parents to spend time with. Go online and join a mom/baby chat group or Facebook Page. The American lifestyle is very busy, parents and childcare workers are challenged to deliver healthy food to children while they financially provide for themselves. During these first few months with your baby, let's choose to shower them with Latch Love!

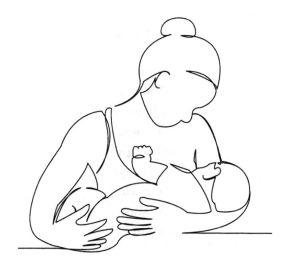

First Mother's Day

New mom
New fun
So blessed
This one
Long nights
Short days
Go Back?
No way.
---author unknown

Chapter 16

Nursing Lifestyle - It's a Big deal, not really!

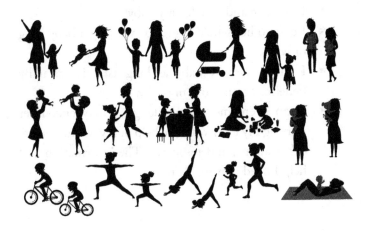

Fit Your Baby Into Your Lifestyle

What do you like to do at home? Do you like to work on your laptop, iPad, SmartPhone. Or do you watch movies or television. Do you spend time in the kitchen catering events or baking? Are you a hairstylist/cosmetologist type, always in the bathroom mirror or are you a gardener, outside tending to flowers? Become a Mama Bear, go bare chested under your robe, for a couple of months. Make a breastfeeding schedule/calendar. What is a "mama bear", remember the story of Goldilocks? Be persistent in staying on your schedule - nursing and expressing milk for your baby. To get more housework done, wear the baby in a sling. With proper planning, nursing can give you more freedom and independence.

Here are some positive affirmations to help encourage you during this time. Ladies, repeat after me -You can do it! ❤

- ★ I am a mother with a new baby that loves me!
- ★ I can love and care for my baby!
- ★ I can do household chores by wearing a baby sling or wrap.
- ★ I will nurse my baby as long as it is mutually beneficial to me and my baby.
- ★ I can overcome any challenges I may encounter nursing my baby with the help of my doctor, nurse, other moms, and resources. The information and help I need is available to me!

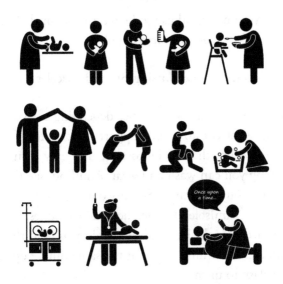

New Mom Fashion

Layer your tops. Twin sweater sets, tank tops and cami tops are convenient and comfortable during this time. Invest in a comfortable cotton nursing bra or nursing cami top and absorbent nursing pads. Sweater wraps, and lightweight poncho are very comfortable and useful during this time. Also layering your cloth baby sling, with your outfit - wearing a coordinated baby sling makes sense and leaves your hands free to do other things. The cloth baby sling has extra fabric to cover yourself while you nurse in public. Practice how you are going to nurse in public at home with your breast pump. Practice hooking and unhooking your nursing bra—with one hand. Practice setting up the breast pump. Carry extra batteries and the electrical and car adaptor. Practice sliding your baby in and out of the sling and nursing the baby in the sling. Build up your confidence with dressing comfortably to nurse your baby and using the pump at home before you express milk at work or nurse in public.

Choose a comfortable Nursing Bra and Bracelet

During the time you nurse, depending on your cup size, you want comfort and support. Soft cotton fabric is best. Find a bra that is comfortable and easy to unlatch, something you can wash and wear. And find one that will not make you too warm. Some women prefer a nursing tank top or camisole. Try on the different styles. Are you left handed or right handed? How will you hold the baby and unlatch your nursing bra at the same time. Look for a simple clasp to unsnap.

What is a nursing bracelet? A nursing bracelet is a piece of jewelry moms wear to keep track of what side to nurse the baby. A mom can easily move the bracelet from wrist to wrist to remind the mom to start nursing on the right or left side to prevent engorgement. This bracelet could be given as a gift to the new mom.

Chapter 17

Let down your Emotions – When the Milk Spills!

When things don't go as planned, it's okay to cry. Talk to your family, children and spouse/partner to sort things out - reflect and rest. Talk to a counselor to sort your feelings. Adding a baby to your lifestyle changes your family dynamics.

Situations You May Find Yourself In

- o Father separated from baby
- o Mom separated from baby
- o Identify two caregivers for baby
- o Join at least two online groups/apps
- o Identify medical/support resource
- o Being a single mom
- o Sick baby NICU
- o Sick parent or grandparent in NICU
- o Moving home
  - ✓ Living in temp housing
  - ✓ Starting new job
- o Divorce or Death in Family

Get Your Mind Right

- ✓ Review the positive affirmations in this book
- ✓ Join and connect to online support, social media support
- ✓ Subscribe to text service and download Mom, Baby apps
- ✓ Join Facebook Mom Groups

Stay Positive

- ★ Visit with favorite people
- ★ Keep conversation pleasant and light and truthful-keep it real
- ★ Repeat positive affirmations
- ★ Don't be so hard on yourself, set goals, aim for it, reach it, then repeat. Some goals take longer

Bible Verses for Meditation

Isaiah 66:11
For you will nurse and be satisfied at her comforting breasts; you will drink deeply and delight in her overflowing abundance

1 Peter 2:2
Like newborn babies, crave pure spiritual milk, so that by it you may grow up in your salvation, now that you have tasted tat the Lord is good.

Luke 11:27
As Jesus was saying these things, a woman in the crowd called out, "Blessed is the mother who gave you birth and nursed you."

Being a Preemie Mom

At first I cried, I was terrified.
Then I saw you.
You were still my child, you just came
Sooner that we had planned.
Prematurity they said. NICU they said.
Everything was so different, but again
What hadn't changed is that you were
Still my child, I was still your mom.
If you could do this, so could I.
I don't cry much anymore.
I am a strong preemie mom.
---Preemie Support and Awareness

How can I get more sleep?

To get more rest, place the crib or bassinet beside the bed so you can nurse the baby on your side then place in the bassinet. Nursing at night keeps your milk supply up and facilitates your childbirth recovery process. Following childbirth, let your body heal itself naturally, nursing facilitates the healing process of the uterus. If you are a stay at home mom, nursing at night, means you are nursing 24/7, day and night; it keeps your milk supply up; and gives you the ecological breastfeeding protective effect which may include natural birth control. Always use another birth control method to be safe. Especially if your period has not returned.

- ✓ Nourish yourself by getting adequate rest
- ✓ How many hours of sleep do you need
- ✓ Hire a sitter; ask a family, friend watch baby while you catch up on your sleep!

What does your Health Insurance Cover?

Call your insurance agency about what is covered, visit their website to be sure. Breast pumps are covered. What else? Explore public health assistance; Medicaid has pregnancy coverage, that may cover your newborn for a few weeks after birth. Don't be embarrassed to ask about these topics. Especially if you are a student, single, or new small business owner.

- ❖ Career Counseling Services
- ❖ Health Department

Feed your Infant for Free and Lose Weight

- ❖ Counseling Services
- ❖ Medical care for Baby
- ❖ Breast Pump Rental
- ❖ Babysitting and Child Care Referral
- ❖ Job Placement
- ❖ Housing Assistance

Chapter 18

Mama, I wanna milkie! -Nursing a 2 Year Old and Beyond!

- ✓ Cleanliness
- ✓ Nursing in public
- ✓ Weaning
- ✓ Benefits of extending nursing
- ✓ What is spouse/partner opinion

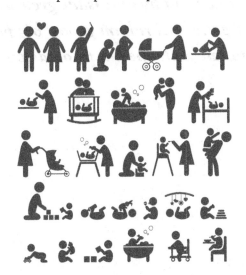

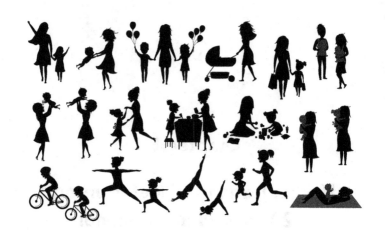

Thinking of Weaning your Baby?

Genesis 21:8
As time went by and Isaac grew and
was weaned, Abraham gave a big party
to celebrate the happy occasion.

A Mother's Prayer

Dear Lord
It's such a hectic day
Yet when I steal a moment, Lord,
Just at the sink or ironing board,
To ask the blessing of your Grace,
I see then in my small one's face.
That you have blessed me all the while-
As I stoop to kiss THAT precious smile!
---Author Unknown

Chapter 19

Field Trips with Baby – 20 Dates with Baby!

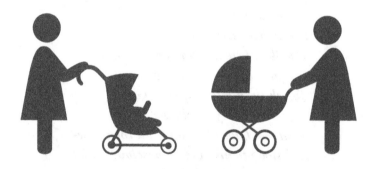

It's time to get out of the house. Explore and rediscover the world with your new baby!!

There's vitamin D outside! Sunshine is good for you and the baby! Put the baby in the stroller and push! Take a quick walk outside for a few minutes! A change of scenery and staying active is help adjust to being a new mom!!

The Wheels on the Car Go Round and Round -Traveling in Cars - Road Tripping

- ☐ Play kids music in the car
- ☐ Proper car seat in the car; change as the child grows; take to Fire Department to have it checked
- ☐ Have portable potty in the trunk of the car so we were never rushed; just park in a concealed area
- ☐ Have snacks in car so we would not have to stop get out of car and wait in line at a fast food restaurants or snacks from the gas station.
- ☐ Timed the trip after a meal or after a heavy snack so kids would not be hungry. Packasnack and keep in the trunk of the car.
- ☐ Have afternoon snack ready for kids as soon as they returned home or entered the car before a commute
- ☐ Keep snacks for mom and baby in diaper bag.
- ☐ Use bathroom before riding in a car

Up Up and Away! - Traveling in Airplane

- ☐ Traveling with kids can be challenging, anticipate everything. Carry food, books, and videos/toys.
- ☐ Anticipate sitting confined in the plane- stretch legs, run play, talk loud before you board the plane
- ☐ Get some fresh air, go to the playground/play area
- ☐ Fitness is important - get kids outside and be active - give active playtime before having them to sit down and be quiet.
- ☐ When sitting in an airport - watch movies on iPhone/mobile device

Travel Food

- ✓ Manual breast pump, Formula powder, empty baby bottle/sippy cup, distilled water
- ✓ When traveling cut up fruit and place in Ziploc bags, grapes, cantaloupes, strawberries, crackers, cheese crackers, sandwiches, bottled water and whole grain breads or their favorite foods
- ✓ Food, having a snack and taking a quick walk, helps keep the kids settled when they are full and get a chance to run around, they seem to have better behavior
- ✓ Names on snack bags make it more interesting for the little one and gives them a sense of ownership and responsibility. They seemed to want to hold onto the bags - brown bags are great because they can throw them away.

------------------20 Dates with Your Baby-------------------

1. In the Kitchen/High Chair

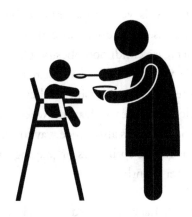

This is a good time to work on manners and playtime!

What to Wear: Clothes with pictures of fruit on them and clothes to get messy!

What to Have: Toys and puzzles before the food is served; Noodles, rice, and green peas in the highchair is alot of fun!

What to Do: Allow child to sample new foods from highchair, listen and watch child for choking and later allergic reactions. Call doctor and advice nurse if necessary. Move highchair close to you. DO NOT leave your child alone in the kitchen in the highchair. Older toddlers and preschool children could help prepare food for meal time, picnic, or grill. They could use a plastic knife to slice soft bananas or soft strawberries for a fruit salad or skewers.

2. The Backyard

Playing outside in the backyard can increase your child's fitness large, gross motor skills.

Outdoor play is very important to being physically healthy. An increase in outdoor play can increase your child's health and decrease childhood obesity. Have breakfast and snack outside with kids. Take watermelon and popsicles outside. There will be no fussing if they drip. Sometimes there is no clean up or easy clean up when you take wet or sticky foods outside. It is also a nice way to calm down after running through the sprinklers or playing kickball in the Spring, Summer months.

What to Wear: Easy wash and wear clothes, closed toe shoes with no-slip soles

What to Pack: Water bottle and light fruit snack for after game

What to Do: Play simple games kids like to play in the backyard such as soccer, dodgeball, hopscotch, splash in the pool or run through the sprinkler.

Plant a Garden:

Establishing a family garden can be a special time with your new baby and older children. Read a story about gardens, go to the grocery or garden center to look at the vegetable that you are about to plant then buy the seeds or the plant.

Plan your garden first to see where to plant the items

for proper spacing for growth. De-weed the garden everyday and draw a picture of the garden with the kids, draw a picture of the front and backyard. The baby can sit in the stroller....and watch you tend the garden!

Allow your children to pick fruit and vegetables from your garden and take inside to cook. Kids can make salads with the tomatoes and greens, they grow. Let them experiment with sauteing or roasting the vegetables they grow, for instance, squash, okra, onions, etc. Work on your garden while a family member grills outside.

3. Doctor's Office

Follow the immunization schedule and well baby doctor visit schedule. Children can learn body awareness at the doctor's office.

What to Wear: Easy off snap or zippered outfits

What to Pack: A blanket for coverage and warmth

Leave this at Home: It is natural to be scared, nervous, or anxious at the doctors office! Relax!

What to Do: Sometimes it's helpful for 2 people to go to the doctor appointment to hold the baby and to listen and speak with the doctor and gather items and console baby while crying. Try to get the baby to stop crying while in the car seat for the ride home. If a child receives immunization and cries and becomes irritable, plan and enjoy a relaxed, easy day after leaving the doctor's office. Do something the calm down the baby.

4. Grocery Store

I want the red cart mommy!

Leave this at Home: Bring your own cover or wipes for shopping cart.

What to Do: Eat, Rest, use the bathroom before you go shopping. Bring a snack for your own child such as water, juice box so they can focus on their own food, not the food on the shelves. Keep the shopping trip short to avoid a meltdown! Keep the baby safe in the cart -remember babies gain weight in just a few weeks and the car seat can move and shift in the cart! Some moms wear their babies in a sling when grocery shopping.

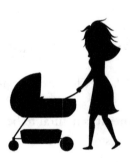

5 . Shopping Mall

Nice social time to share with your baby.

Even though online shopping is popular, go to the mall to try on clothes. Go to the mall during the holidays for Santa, Easter Bunny, holiday performances and art shows. The mall is a good place for a stroller ride! Meet up with other moms and seniors to do laps around the mall. Know where the restroom is if potty training your toddler.

6. Farmer's Market

For parents who want to homeschool, the farmer's market provides a lesson on diet, agriculture and food from different cultures.

What to Wear: Casual shopping clothes

What to Pack: Bring your colorful recycle bags

What to Do: Hold, smell fruit and vegetables; buy small items to puree for baby food

7. Church/Temple

Good time to work on behavior and learn about faith in something other than themselves

What to Do: Pack quiet toys. Like the library, kids have to sit quiet and be still. Learn about history and religion. Talk about values and family. Find a family oriented church, faith hall!

8. Family Restaurant

Don't stay too long in the restaurant. Try to keep the area around you clean. Bring lots of patience and high tolerance level. Go to restaurant on kids eat free night so their noise and energy level can match the atmosphere. Be ready to cut food in bite sizes. If available ask for high chairs or toddler seats.

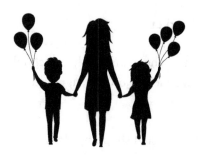

9. Street Festival (Music, Art)

Great time for a social studies lesson for the homeschoolers. Wear bright colored, art gear. Sing along, dance! If it is a city park, bring blanket and snacks for a picnic with live music. Most street events require walking so keep the stroller light. If the festival is family friendly go early before the crowds are too thick for strollers. It's always fun to visit the vendor tables. Wear your baby in a sling!

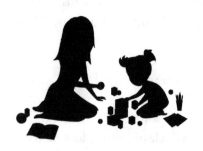

10. Playground

Nice social time to share with your baby and it allows them to practice body movement and fitness.

What to Wear: Kids can wear lightweight cotton shorts, closed toe shoes with rubber, non slip soles,

What to Pack: Use of a double stroller: convenience of having two kids riding side by side, lightweight umbrella stroller is easy to collapse and place in trunk. Kids can take turns pushing each other and hang a bag of snacks or half pint of water stroller, while riding.

What to Do: Have a snack in the car for after playground; Snacks can be placed in a soft, cooler bag. Snacks such as cantaloupe, crackers, nuts, banana. Drink water after playtime so you don't have to use the bathroom. .Check the playground for safety for appropriate age level for child. Check playground equipment for sharp edges. Try to prevent pinched fingers on the swings.

11. Pet Store

Animal and care taking lessons for child happen here! Many child like to watch dogs being groomed. Start planning for buying a family pet. Be alert and keep your baby close to you if she is afraid of dogs and cats. Some kids get excited and point and scream at the animals as they move around. Go to the pet store on rescue day to see more animals. Take your time when you go so you will have time to observe the animals. Go to the pet store with an idea of what kind of animal or breed you may like.

12. Zoo

Nice time to learn about animals, climate/weather, and geography. Look for animal babies, watch the animals eat lunch and care for their young! Let your baby, toddler bring their animal cards, books, and toys. Pack a snack in a soft, cooler bag and watch the animals prowl.

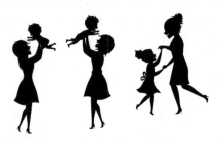

13. Mommy & Me Music Group

What to Wear: Comfortable clothes to dance, and sit on the floor

What to Pack: A fresh fruit snack for after class

Leave this at Home: Bad attitude, music will uplift your mood!

What to Do: Play music as an activity, use the CD, soundtrack from class during your everyday routines, Play your child's favorite song to signal a certain time/event --play

Barney Song to signal clean up time, music can be used to entertain children while it is raining outside and can't go outside to play, music can calm children for bedtime, music can help children in the morning - getting them energized for school, music can make tub time or bathroom time more fun. Shake, shake, shake, play music at home or in car. Give your baby, lots of laughter and love here! Let them try different music instruments!

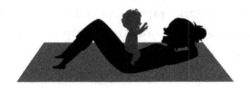

14. Mommy & Me Gymnastics

Take your child somewhere where they can run and jump and leap. People live in small spaces. Go to the jumping parks! Let your child do jumping jacks, cartwheels, forward rolls. Trampoline parks are great for rainy, cold, days. Bounce and jump!

15. Library/Storytime

Reading a story with your child is so special. Favorite places in the house to read a story are books in bed and reading in the bathroom during tub time.

What to Wear: Comfortable Clothes that you can sit on floor

What to Pack: Return library books, School/Summer Grade Level Reading Lists

Leave this at Home: Food-no food and drinks in the library; bad behavior

What to Do: Reading aloud, take turns reading pages, and talking about the pictures; Read Magazines-Kids Magazine, Hidden Pictures, I Spy. You can nurse your infant while reading to their sibling. When you read to your child be expressive - use facial expressions and inflection of voice. Reading can calm baby down before nap and meal time. Is the talking cow here today?

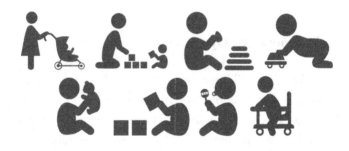

16. Children's Art Museum

I want to paint today!
Good place for socialization and mental stimulation for your child!

What to Wear: Art gear

What to Pack: Pack light

What to Do: Take time to look at the art, the details of the activities, talk aloud and ask questions about what the activity or event.

17. Walking Trail

Excellent time and place for a science lesson and time for peaceful meditation. Walking along the creek, trail, mountain and hilltop is a popular escape or retreat from hectic days of traffic commutes.

What to Wear: Comfortable athletic gear, jogging stroller

What to Pack: Pedometer, phone, keys

Leave this at Home: Leave food in car, don't litter, carry sunglasses.

What to Do: Be careful outside, enjoy the sunshine, gaze upwards towards the clouds in the sky, the tree line, while you walk, talk some and walk quietly to hear the sounds of nature. Take scenic pictures.

18. Car Road Trip to Visit Family/Friends

Visiting family members teaches family priority, and family support! Trips during the holiday are special. Going to big football games and school band competitions are especially thrilling and can be mini reunions!

What to Wear: Comfortable layered outfit;

What to Pack: New, Different Toys they don't play with-

Leave this at Home: Too many pillows, too many snacks

What to Do: Don't pack car too tight, leave space in and around seats, make frequent bathroom, leg stretch breaks. Take a walk, get fresh air and sunshine when you get out the car.

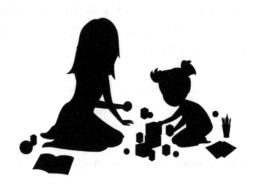

19. Plane Trip to Visit Family/Friends

This is another time to visit the map and have a lesson in geography

What to Wear: Comfortable walking shoes, lightweight stroller

What to Pack: Snacks, quiet toys

Leave this at Home: Pack light, take items that may get lost or left behind

What to Do: Watch planes, people in uniforms-pilots, flight attendants, security guards, watch the sights and hear the sounds of the airport!

20. Kids Movie Matinee

Excellent time and place for a kids playdate with their older siblings (elementary/middle school). Summer is a great time for outdoor movies and toddlers can run around or take a nap in the stroller. Kids can wear clothes they can spill food on; shoes that can get sticky! Sit and watch the movie if it isn't too loud for little ears.

Chapter 20

Discussion Guide for Book Club

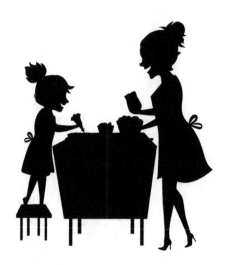

Book Club Topics

- ✓ Daycare/School concerns
- ✓ Join church or faith community
- ✓ Hard day with the baby
- ✓ Easy day with the baby

✓ Planning Date Night
✓ Staying active
✓ Finding a Babysitter
✓ Adjusting to Life with a new baby
✓ Adjusting to Sleep Changes
✓ Adjusting after Divorce or Death in Family
✓ Home Schooling
✓ Job Search/Career Change
✓ Starting a Business
✓ Applying to School
✓ Living in a Multi-generational Home Setting (Baby, parents, grandparents)
✓ Traveling Spouse/Partner Not at Home
✓ Mom in Careers (Military, Law, Business, Medical, Media)
✓ Maintaining your Marriage Relationship

Hire a babysitter to watch children under the age of 5, in another room, for the 2 hour Book Club Discussion.

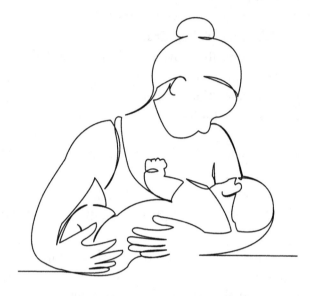

Mother's Heart Poem
I loved you from the very start,
You stole my breath, embraced my heart.
Our life together has just begun
You've part of me my little one.

As mother with child, each day I grew,
My mind was filled with thoughts of you.
I would daydream of the things we would share,
Like late-night bottles and Teddy bears.
--Unknown

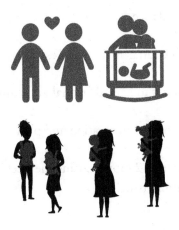

*Discussion Guide for New Mom's
Groups/Ladies Book Clubs
Suggested Agenda*

Welcome and Offer Refreshments

Greeting- Support Group for Moms -Safe environment to share/non judgemental

Loving your new baby

Out and About with Baby - Share good days and bad days

Breastfeeding Support

Weight Loss and Diet Support

Communicating/Partner Relationships

Feed your Infant for Free and Lose Weight

Family Work Balance

Moments of Encouragement and Testimony

Sharing Resources to Meet Personal and Family Goals

---Exchange contact information and plan next meeting--

Reach out to at least 2 moms during the week with the same age child or family issue!

References

In 2011, Regina Benjamin, US Surgeon General, released a Call to Action to Support Breastfeeding. In 2017, the World Health Organization released a publication which states they actively promote breastfeeding as the best source of nourishment for infants and young children.

Here are a few resources to review online.

Let's Move, American Academy of Pediatrics, healthychildren.org, La Leche League, US General Surgeon, American Medical Association, National Medical Association, Choosemyplate.gov, USDA, Food and Drug Administration (FDA),National Association for the Education of Young Children (NAEYC)

Printed in the United States
By Bookmasters